The
Alien Spacebaby's
Dreambook

*...when I close my eyes,
it all comes back.*

S. Glover

ISBN: 978-1-7988-3085-7

ACKNOWLEDGMENTS

Special thanks to Nu and D. for their encouragement, unremitting tolerance, and good humor. Also, a big thank you goes out to all the humans who crossed my path in the murky depths of 28805, messed with my dreamlife, and thus helped to make this project possible.

FORWARD

Many people say that they are unable to remember their dreams. Some even claim that they do not dream at all; but, of course, they do. For some reason, most humans never actively, consciously attempt to impact their dreams whilst awake.

Look at an image in this book for a few minutes before you sleep. Think about it; let your mind wander. Immediately upon awakening, write your dream(s) on the page next to the image. You may well not dream about the image in a *literal* sense – no one can tell what you may see and experience! If you are reluctant to document or divulge your dreamlife, enjoy writing a tale that you think the alien spacebaby might have dreamt after looking at a picture in her book. Or, look at the book with a child and have them tell you their story about each image. Then, take some time to compare and discuss with your friends – so much better than the blue screen life.

Sweet dreams!

<u>*Dreamdate #1 – October Song*</u>

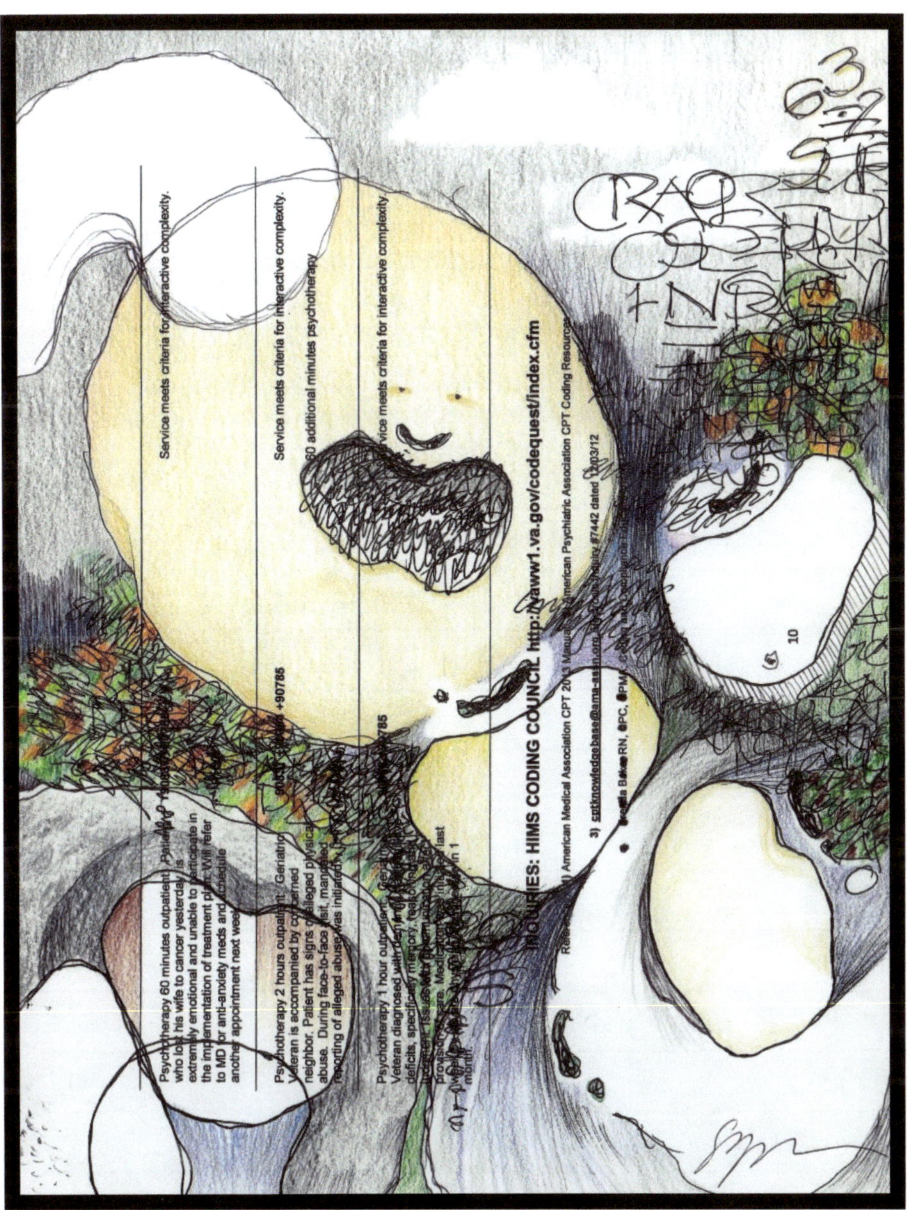
Service meets criteria for interactive complexity.
Service meets criteria for interactive complexity.
30 additional minutes psychotherapy
Service meets criteria for interactive complexity.
Psychotherapy 60 minutes outpatient. Patient is a WWII Veteran who lost his wife to cancer yesterday. He is extremely emotional and unable to participate in the implementation of treatment plan. Will refer to MD for anti-anxiety meds and schedule another appointment next week.
Psychotherapy 2 hours outpatient. Geriatric Veteran is accompanied by concerned neighbor. Patient has signs of alleged physical abuse. During face-to-face visit, mandated reporting of alleged abuse was initiated.
Psychotherapy 1 hour outpatient. Geriatric Veteran diagnosed with dementia. Patient has deficits, specifically memory, reaction time.
INQUIRIES: HIMS CODING COUNCIL http://vaww1.va.gov/codequest/index.cfm
American Medical Association CPT Coding Resource
3) cptknowledgebase@ama-assn.org
RN, CPC, CPMA

Dreamdate #2 – Harvest

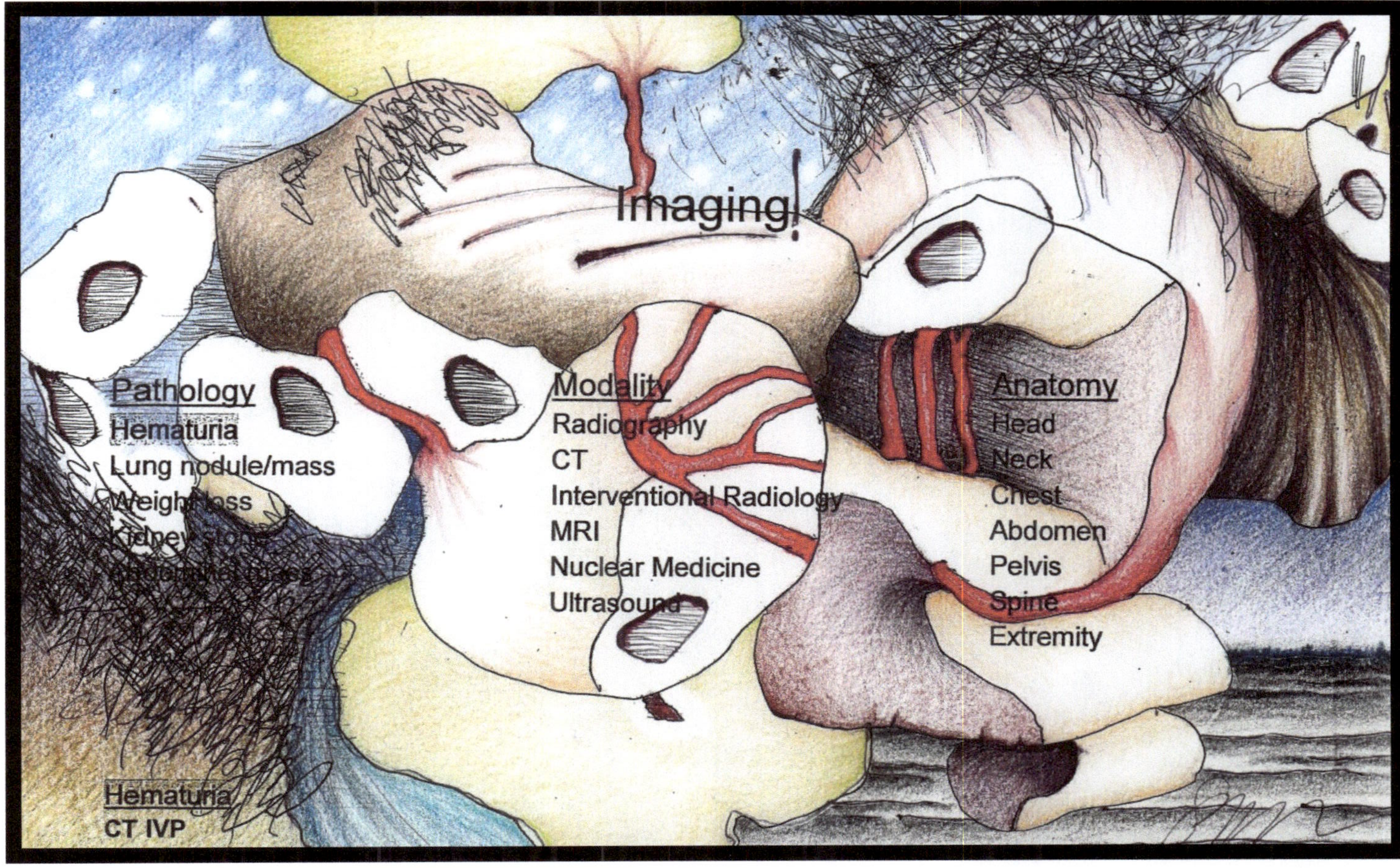
Imaging!
Pathology
Hematuria
Lung nodule/mass
Weight loss
Kidney stone
Modality
Radiography
CT
Interventional Radiology
MRI
Nuclear Medicine
Ultrasound
Anatomy
Head
Neck
Chest
Abdomen
Pelvis
Spine
Extremity
Hematuria
CT IVP

Dreamdate #3 – Hateful

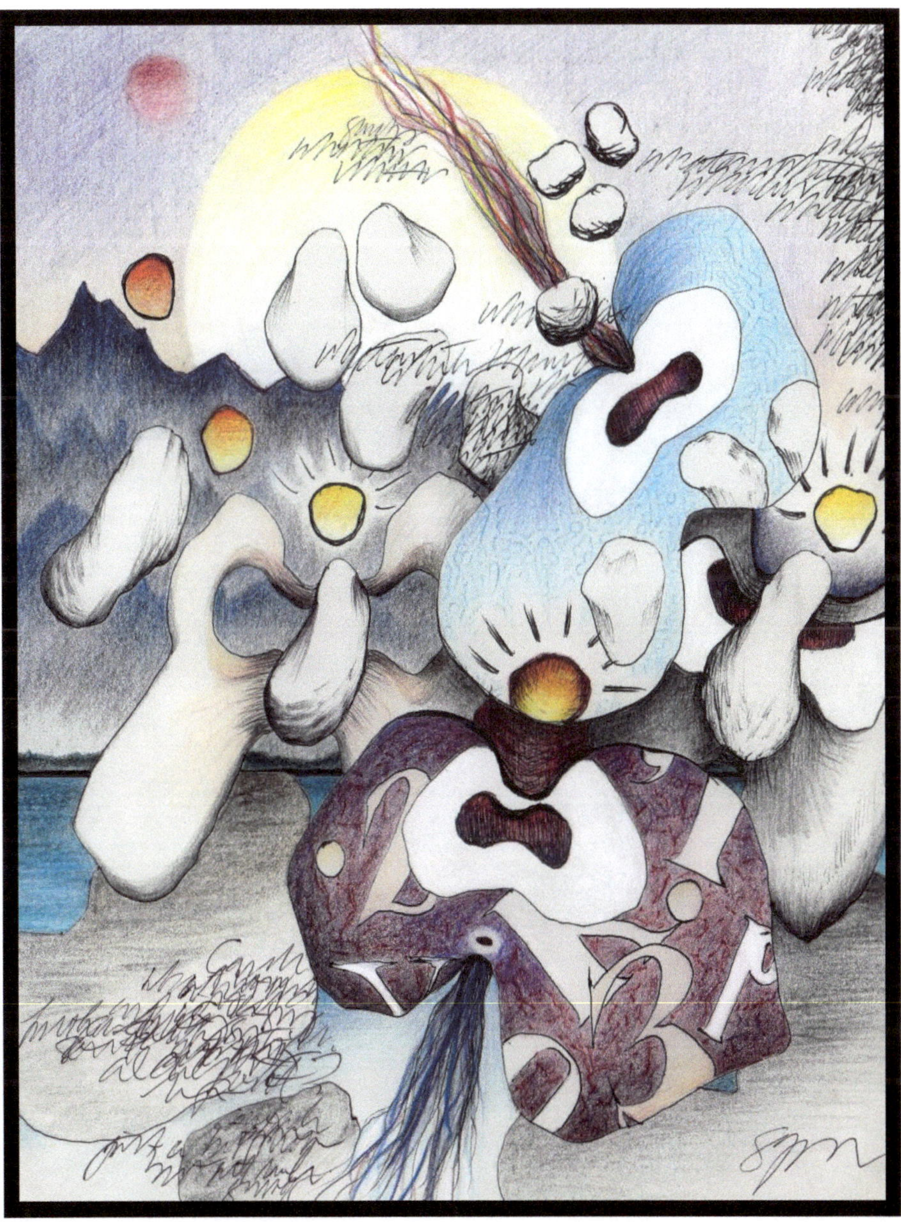

Dreamdate #4 – Vista

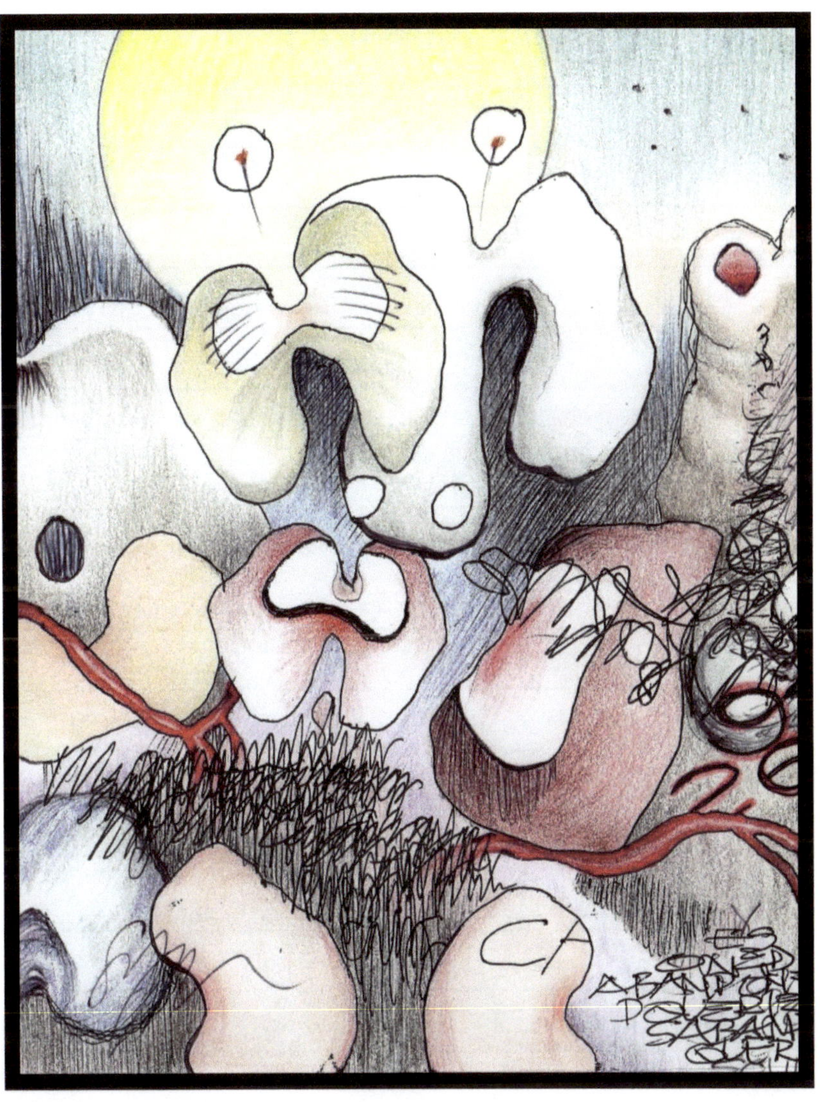

Dreamdate #5 – Summer Bugs

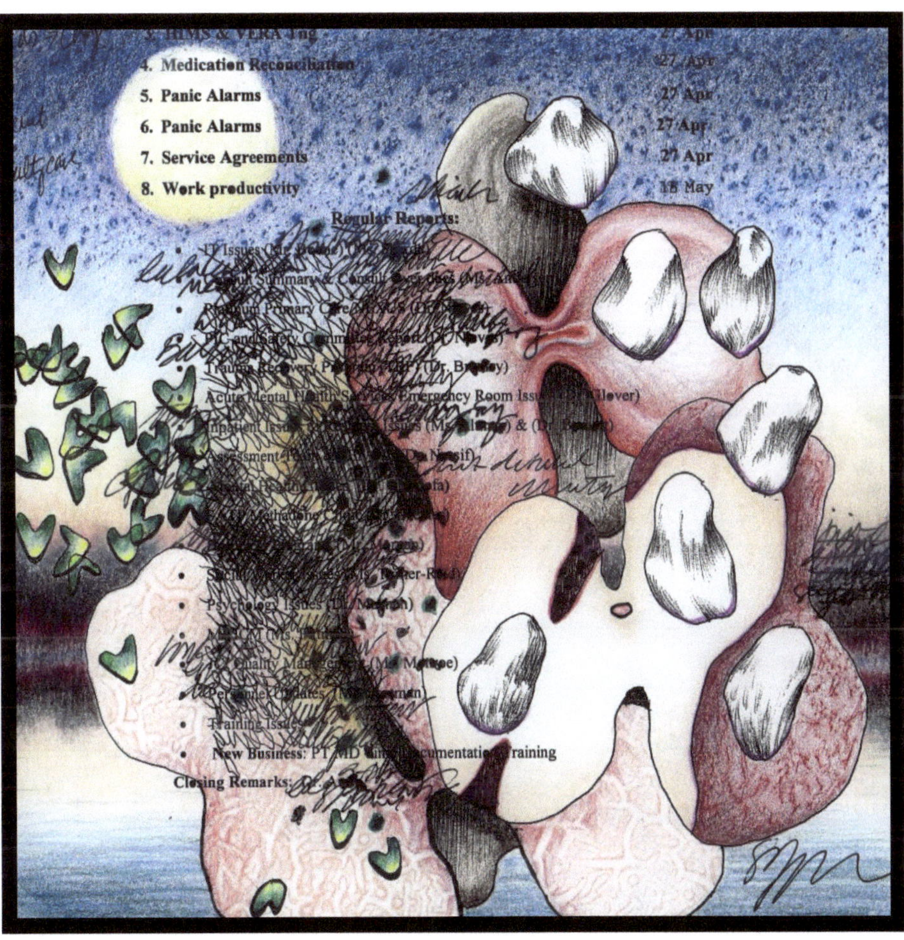
3. HIMS & VERA Tng   27 Apr
4. Medication Reconciliation   27 Apr
5. Panic Alarms   27 Apr
6. Panic Alarms   27 Apr
7. Service Agreements   27 Apr
8. Work productivity   18 May
Regular Reports:
IT Issues
Medical Summary & Consult Services (MSTAR)
Platinum Primary Care (PACTS)
PIC and Safety Committee Report (Dr. Neves)
Trauma Recovery Program (Dr. Bradley)
Acute Mental Health Services/Emergency Room Issues (Dr. Hoover)
Inpatient Issues (MS. Adams) & (Dr.
Assessment (Dr. Nassif)
Mental Health (Dr. Moustafa)
OTP Methadone Clinic
Suicide Prevention (Butler-Reyes)
Psychology Issues (Dr. Newton)
MST
Utilization/Quality Management (Ms. Monroe)
Personnel Updates (Ms. Newman)
Training Issues
New Business: PT/MD Clinic Documentation Training
Closing Remarks:

Dreamdate #6 – Change

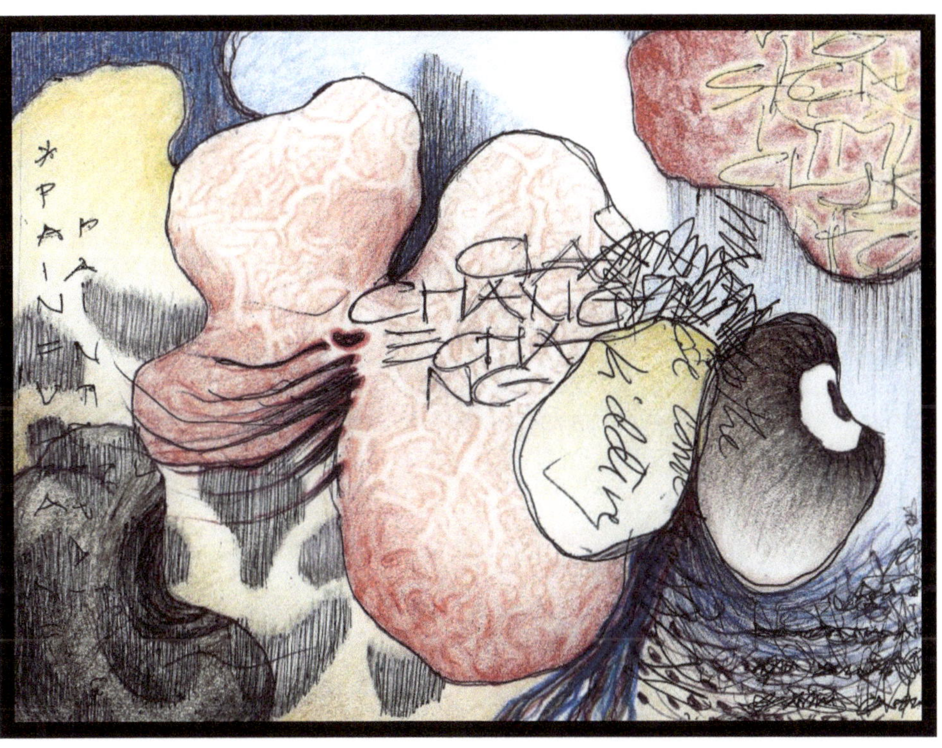

*PAINP
PAINT
CHANGE
CHX
NG

Dreamdate #7 – The Circus Below

2/25/2013

2013 Mental Health CPT
Code Updates

What's Being Changed?
Psychiatric Diagnostic Interview
Individual Psychotherapy
Medication Management
New Codes for Interactive Complexity and
Psychotherapy for Crisis

ALL CPT CODE CHANGES ARE EFFECTIVE
JANUARY 1, 2013

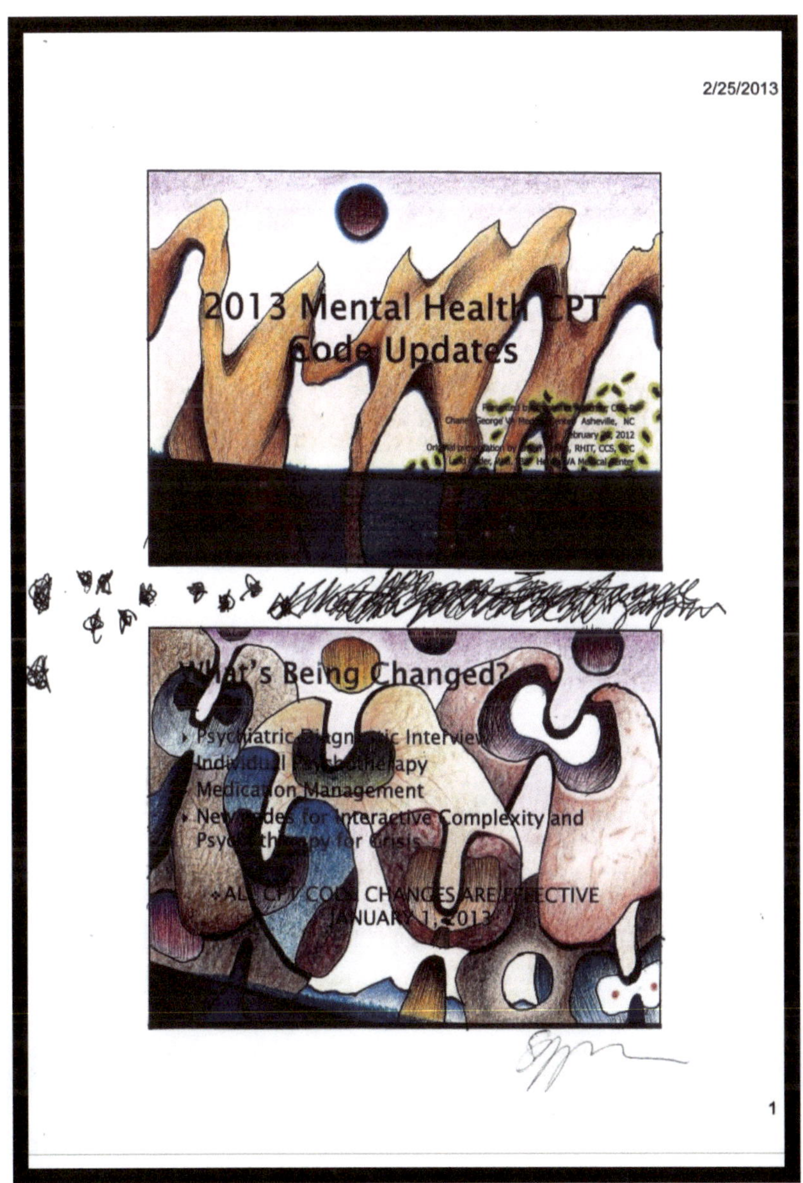

1

<u>Dreamdate #8 – Blue Moon</u>

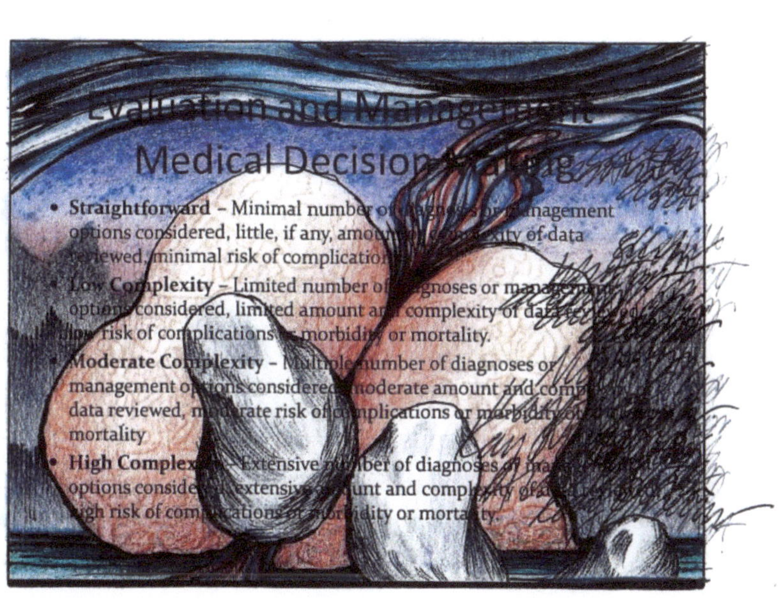

Evaluation and Management
Medical Decision Making
• Straightforward – Minimal number of diagnoses or management options considered, little, if any, amount or complexity of data reviewed, minimal risk of complications
• Low Complexity – Limited number of diagnoses or management options considered, limited amount and complexity of data reviewed, low risk of complications or morbidity or mortality.
• Moderate Complexity – Multiple number of diagnoses or management options considered, moderate amount and complexity of data reviewed, moderate risk of complications or morbidity or mortality
• High Complexity – Extensive number of diagnoses or management options considered, extensive amount and complexity of data reviewed, high risk of complications or morbidity or mortality.

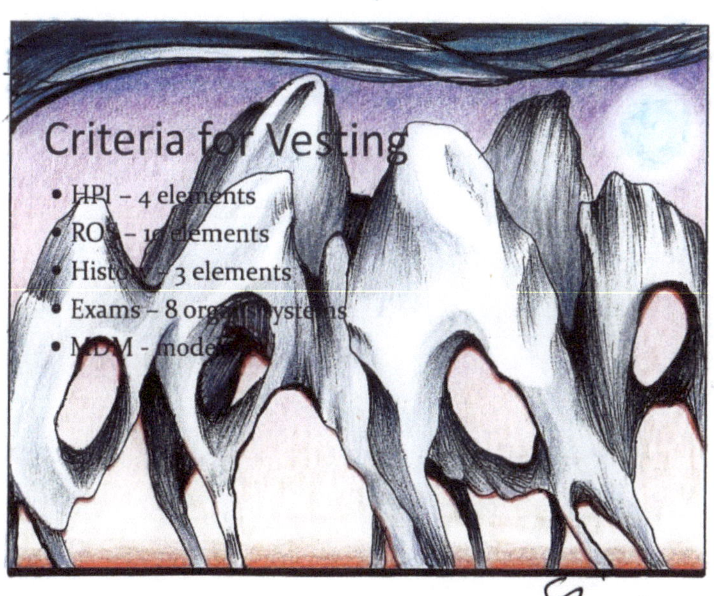

Criteria for Vesting
• HPI – 4 elements
• ROS – 10 elements
• History – 3 elements
• Exams – 8 organ systems
• MDM – moderate

Dreamdate #9 – Butterflies

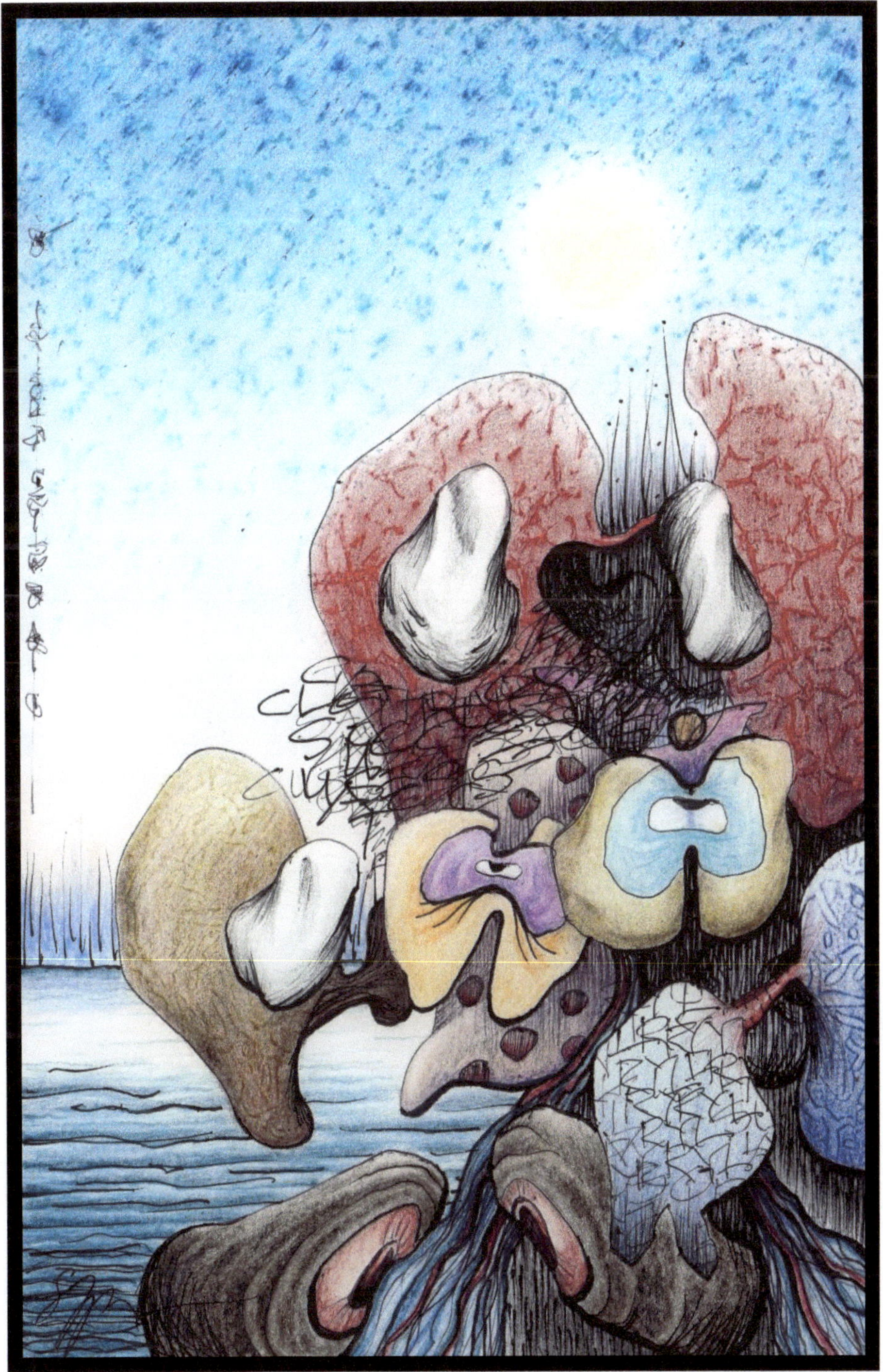

<u>Dreamdate #10 – Excess Baggage</u>

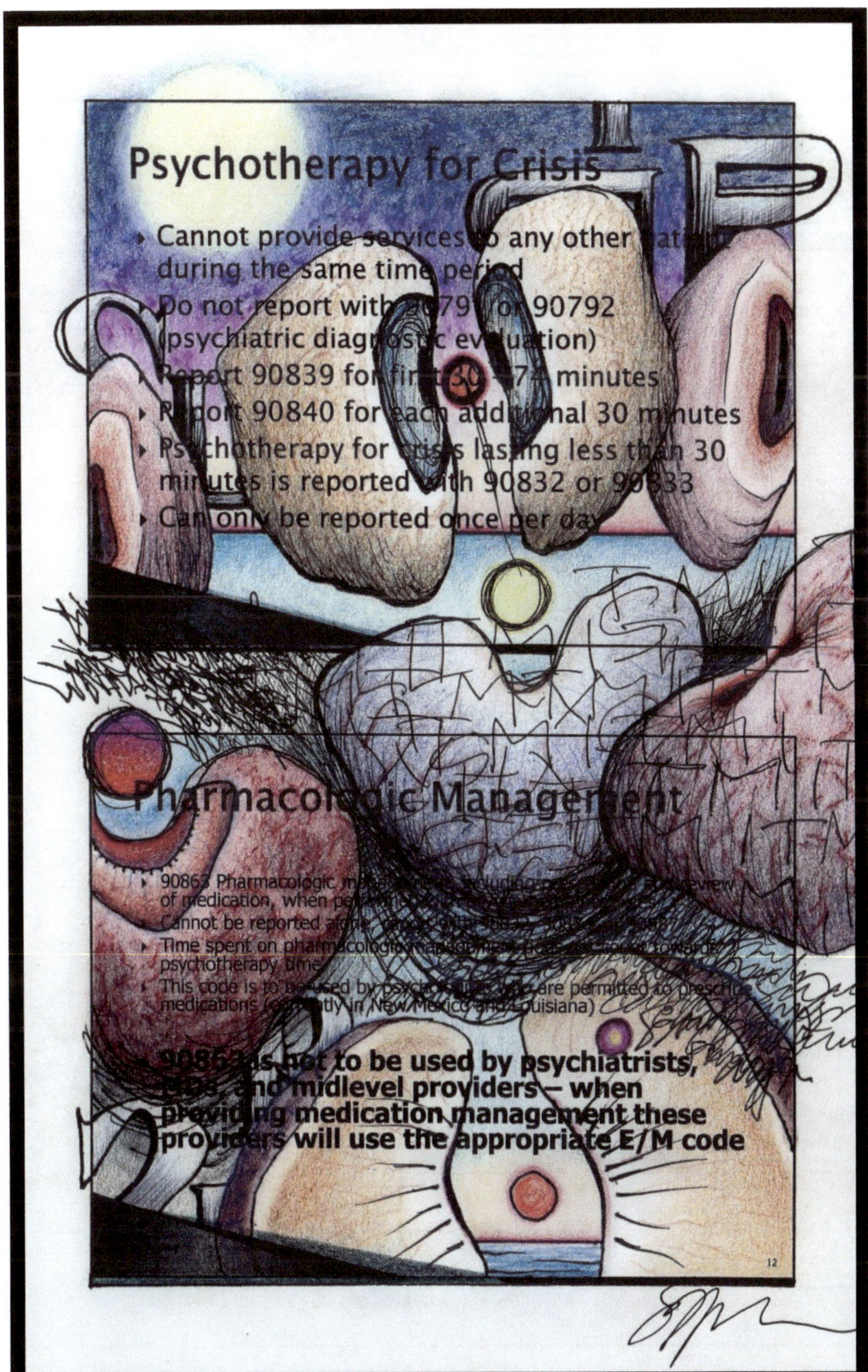

Psychotherapy for Crisis

• Cannot provide services to any other patient during the same time period
• Do not report with 90791 or 90792 (psychiatric diagnostic evaluation)
• Report 90839 for first 30-74 minutes
• Report 90840 for each additional 30 minutes
• Psychotherapy for crisis lasting less than 30 minutes is reported with 90832 or 90833
• Can only be reported once per day

Pharmacologic Management

• 90863 Pharmacologic management, including prescription and review of medication, when performed with psychotherapy services
• Cannot be reported alone, along with 90832, 90834, 90837
• Time spent on pharmacologic management does not count towards psychotherapy time
• This code is to be used by psychologists who are permitted to prescribe medications (currently in New Mexico and Louisiana)

• 90863 is not to be used by psychiatrists, NPPs, and midlevel providers — when providing medication management these providers will use the appropriate E/M code

<u>Dreamdate #11 – Crooked Lake</u>

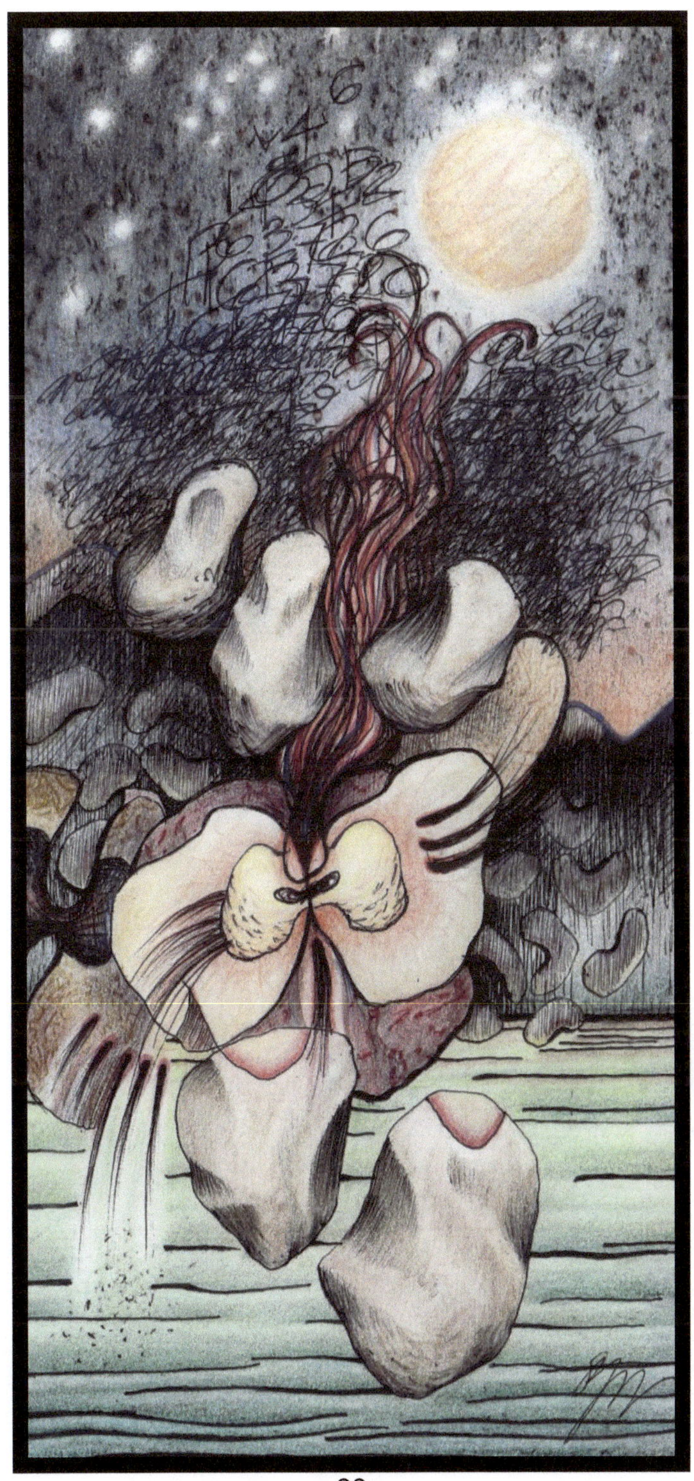

Dreamdate 12 – Pestilence

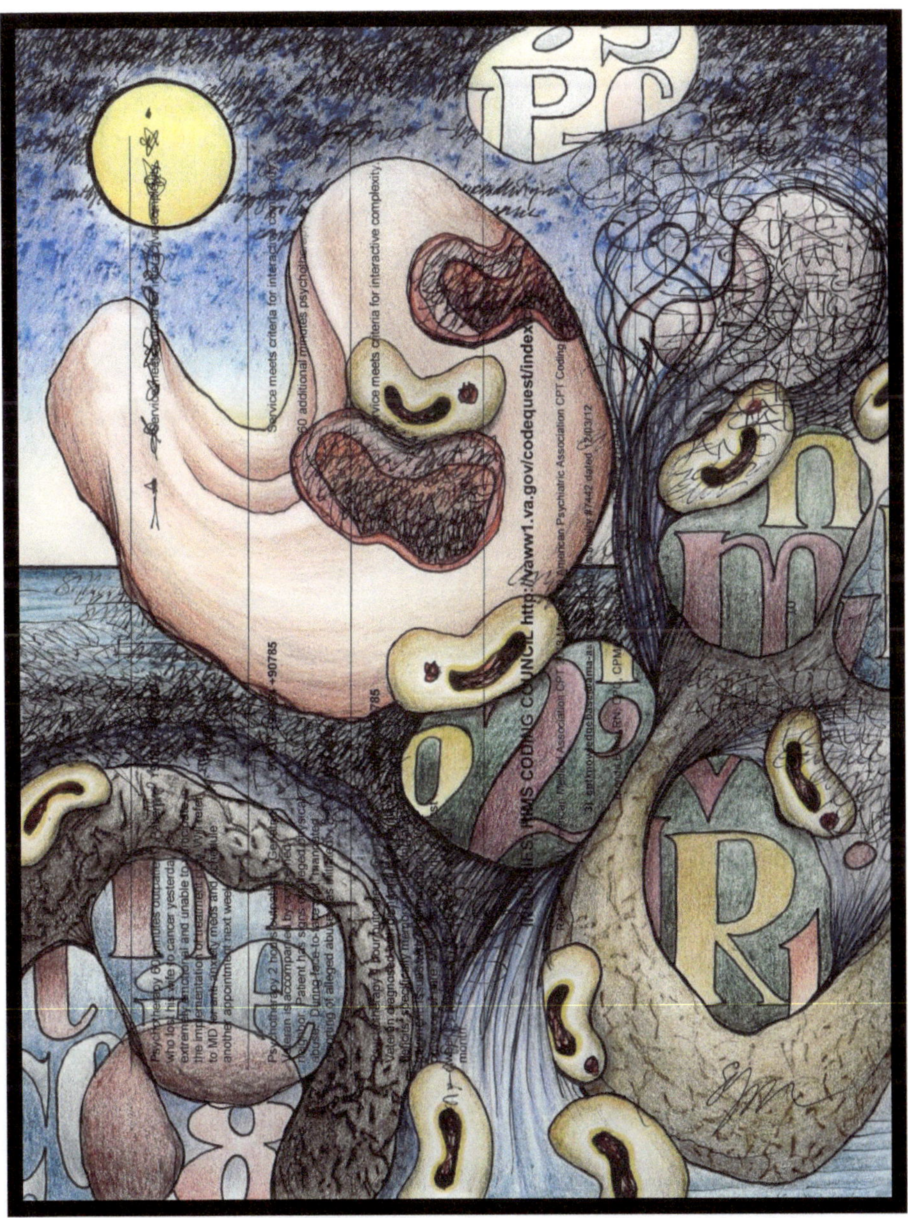

Dreamdate #13 – March Snow

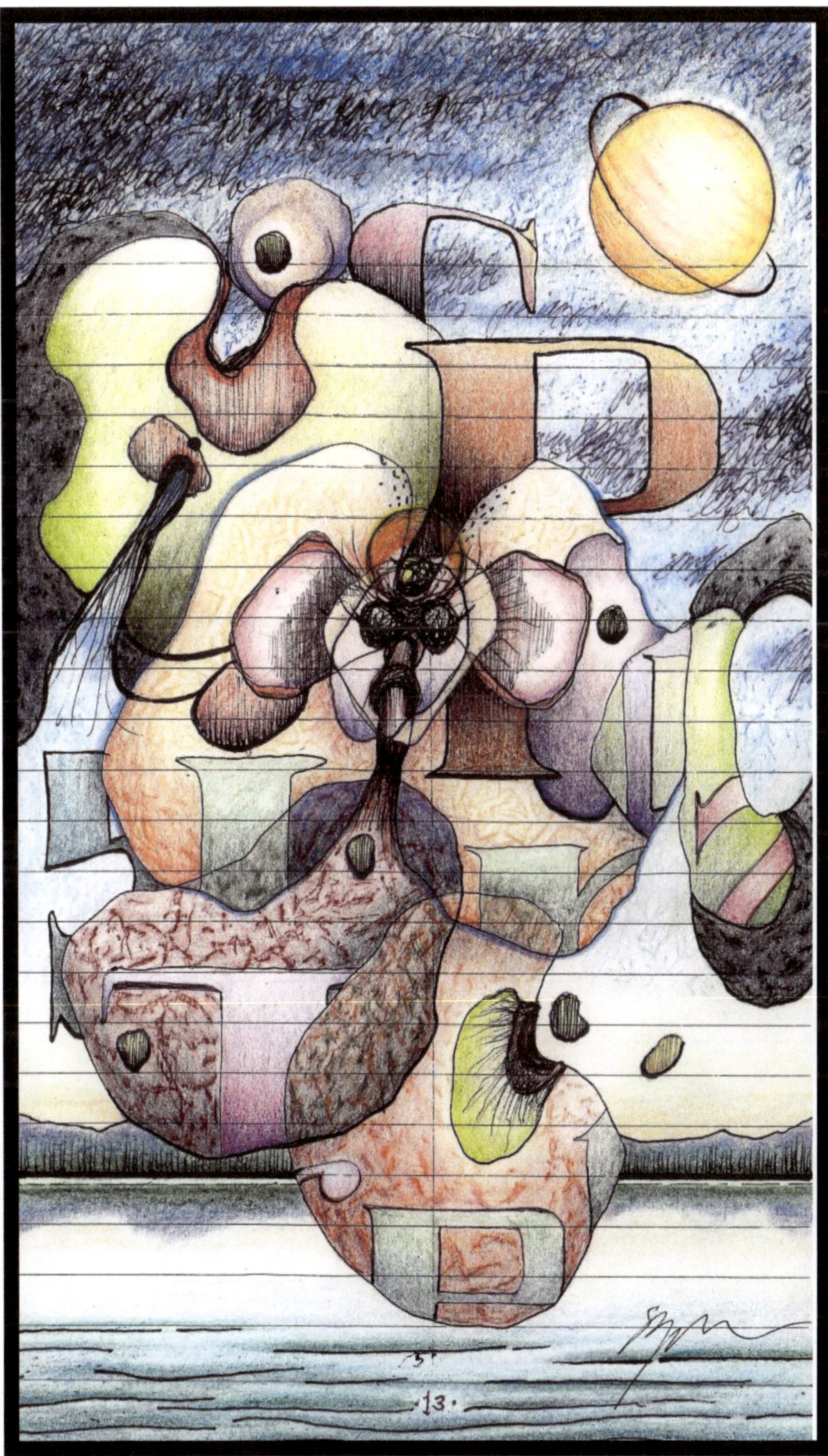

Dreamdate #14 – Pods

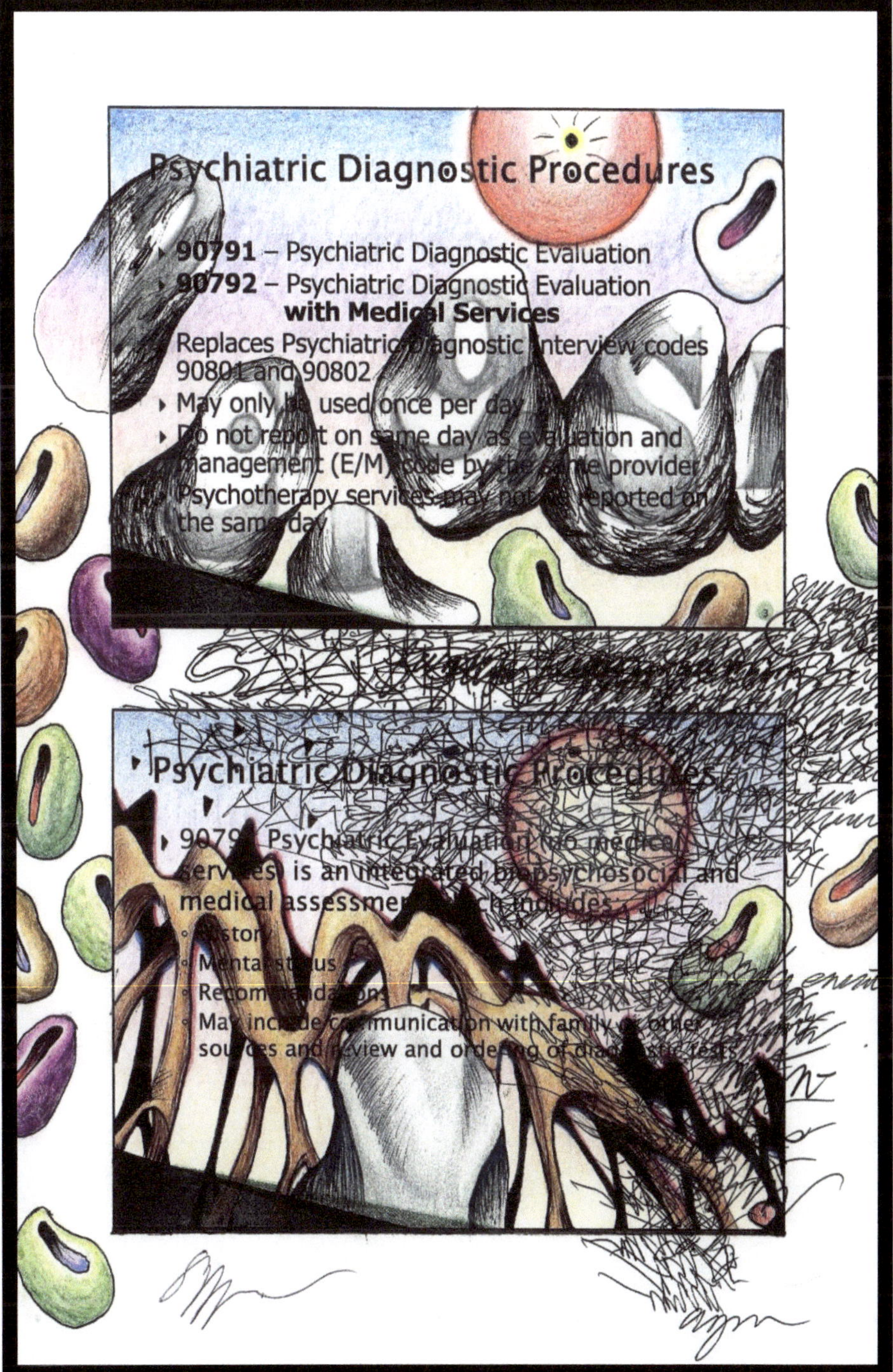
Psychiatric Diagnostic Procedures

90791 – Psychiatric Diagnostic Evaluation
90792 – Psychiatric Diagnostic Evaluation
with Medical Services
Replaces Psychiatric Diagnostic Interview codes
90801 and 90802
May only be used once per day
Do not report on same day as evaluation and
management (E/M) code by the same provider
Psychotherapy services may not be reported on
the same day

Psychiatric Diagnostic Procedures

90791 Psychiatric Evaluation (no medical
services) is an integrated biopsychosocial and
medical assessment which includes:
History
Mental status
Recommendations
May include communication with family or other
sources and review and ordering of diagnostic tests

Dreamdate #15 – Fakery

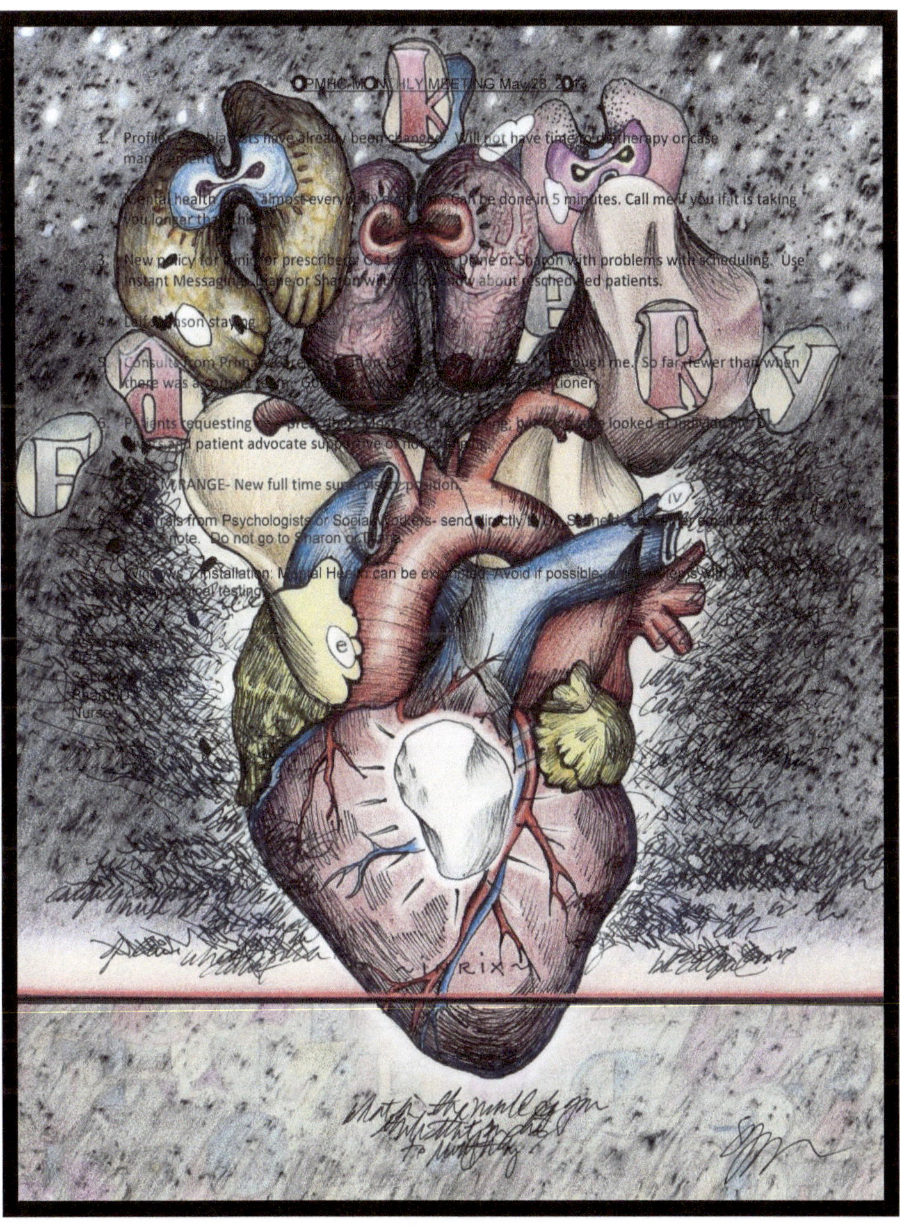
OPMHC MONTHLY MEETING May 28, 2013

Dreamdate #16 – Upriver

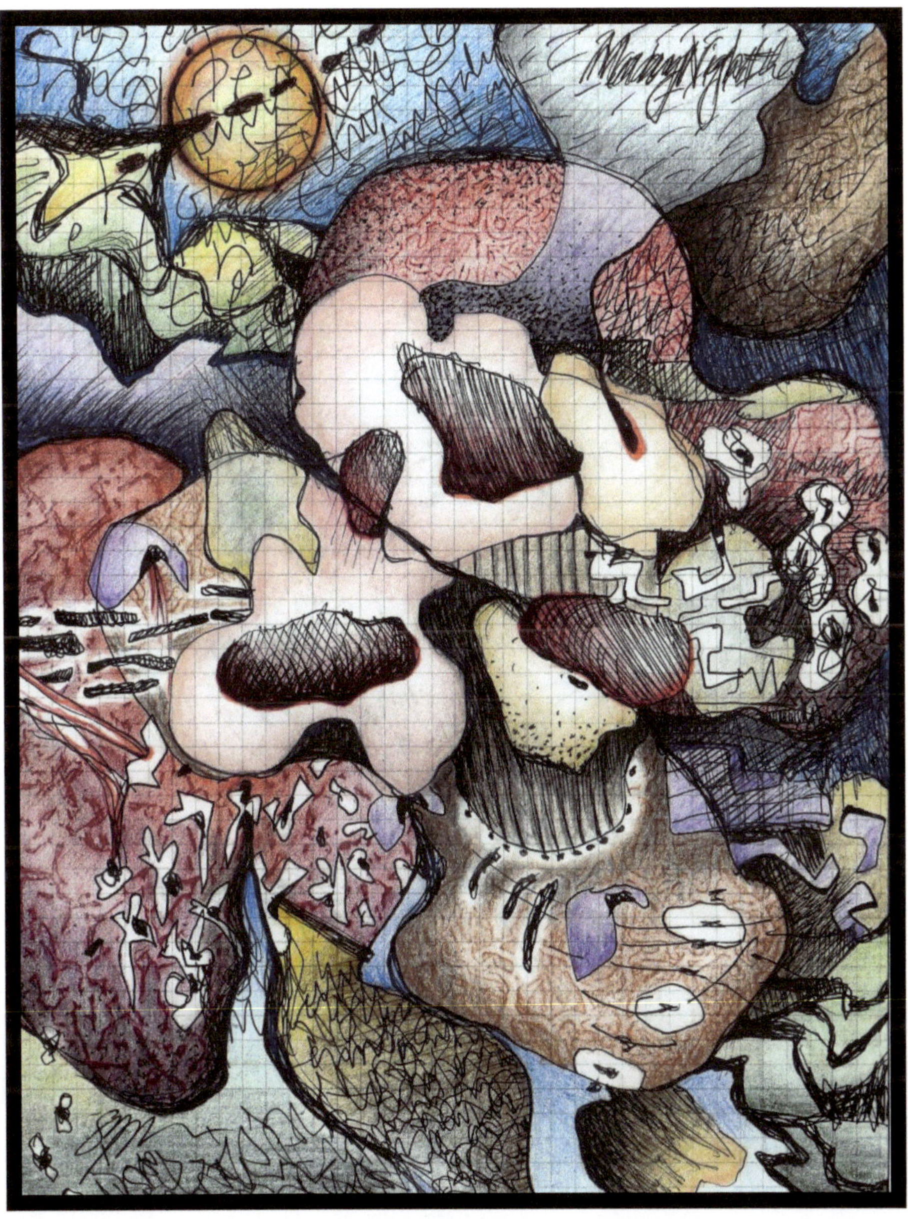
ManyNyght

Dreamdate #17 – Seventeen Again

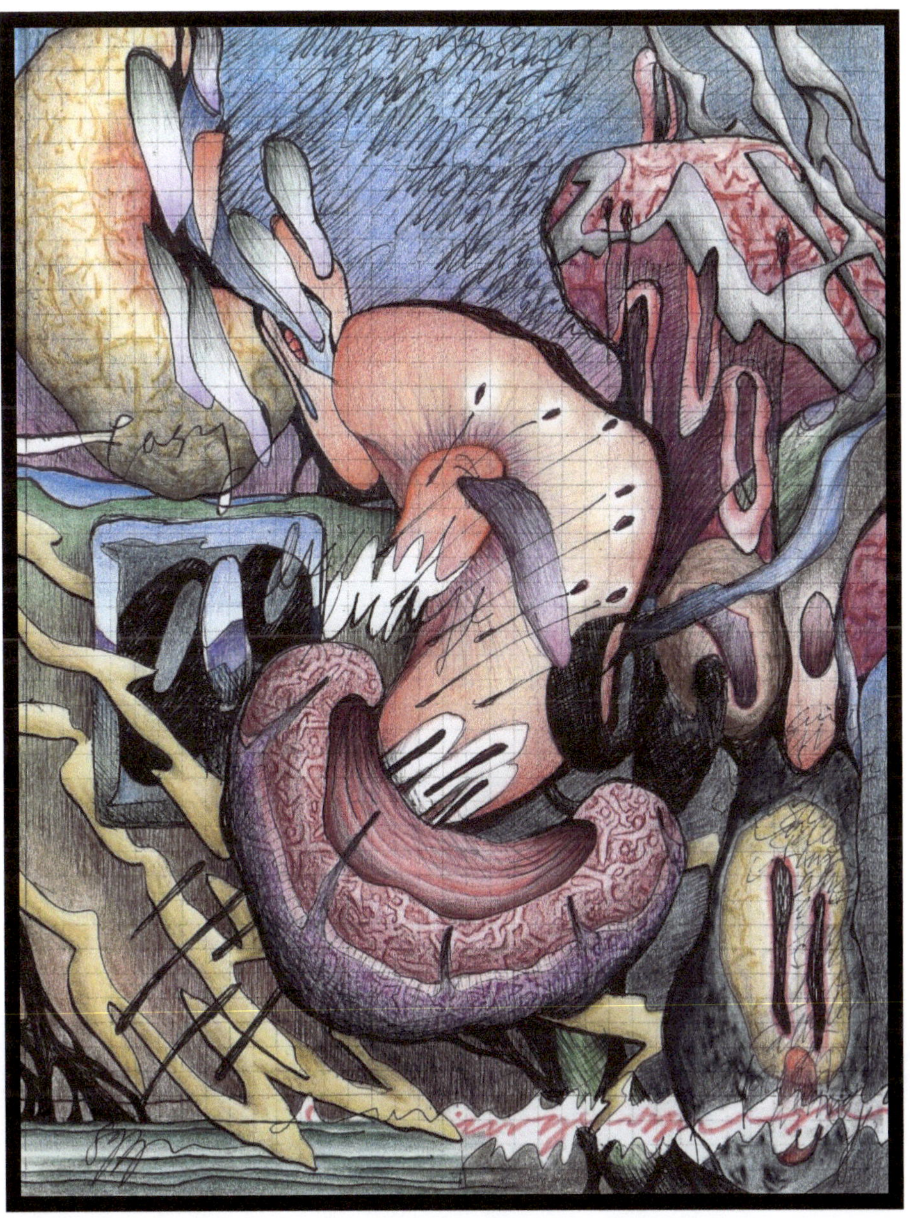

Dreamdate #18 – Across the Bridge

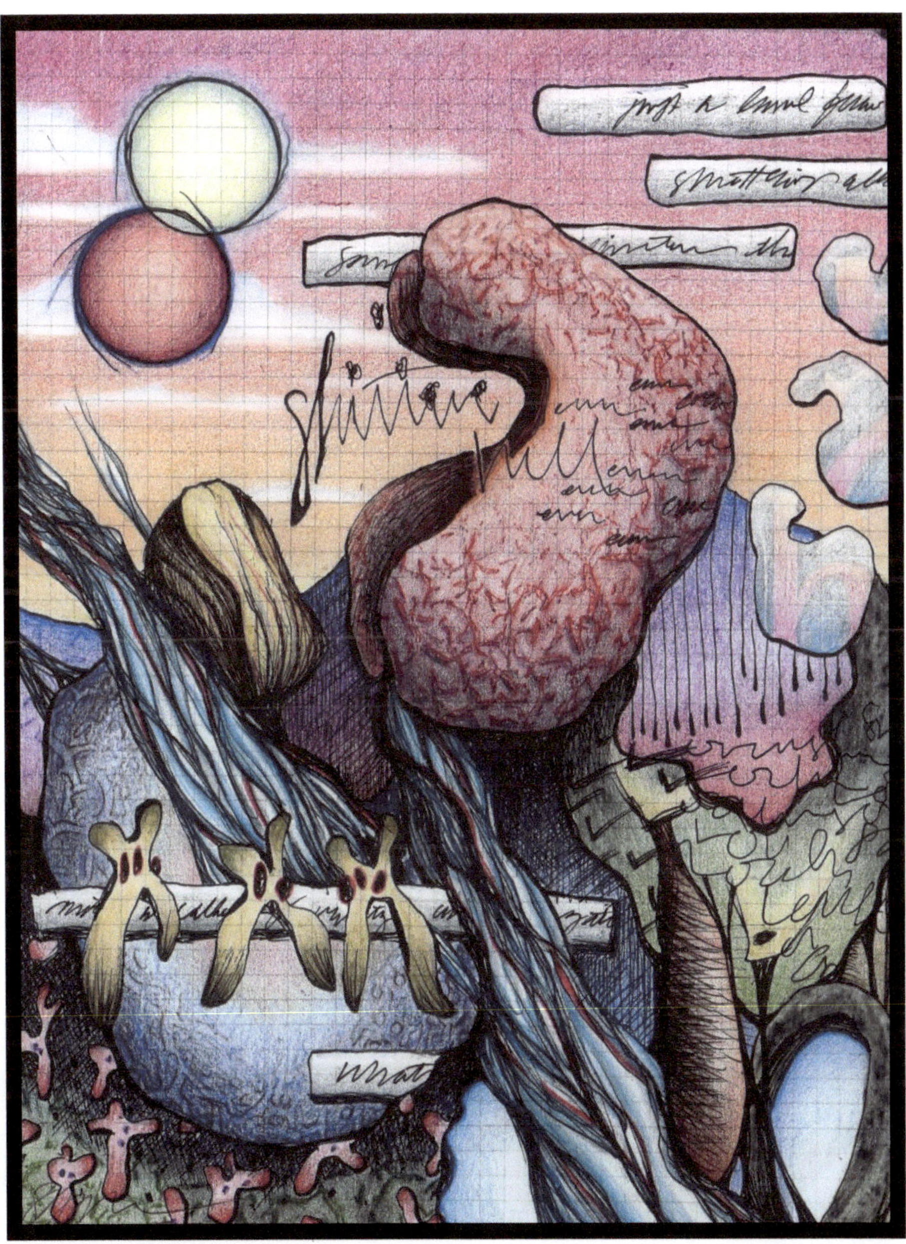

Dreamdate 19 – Blirk

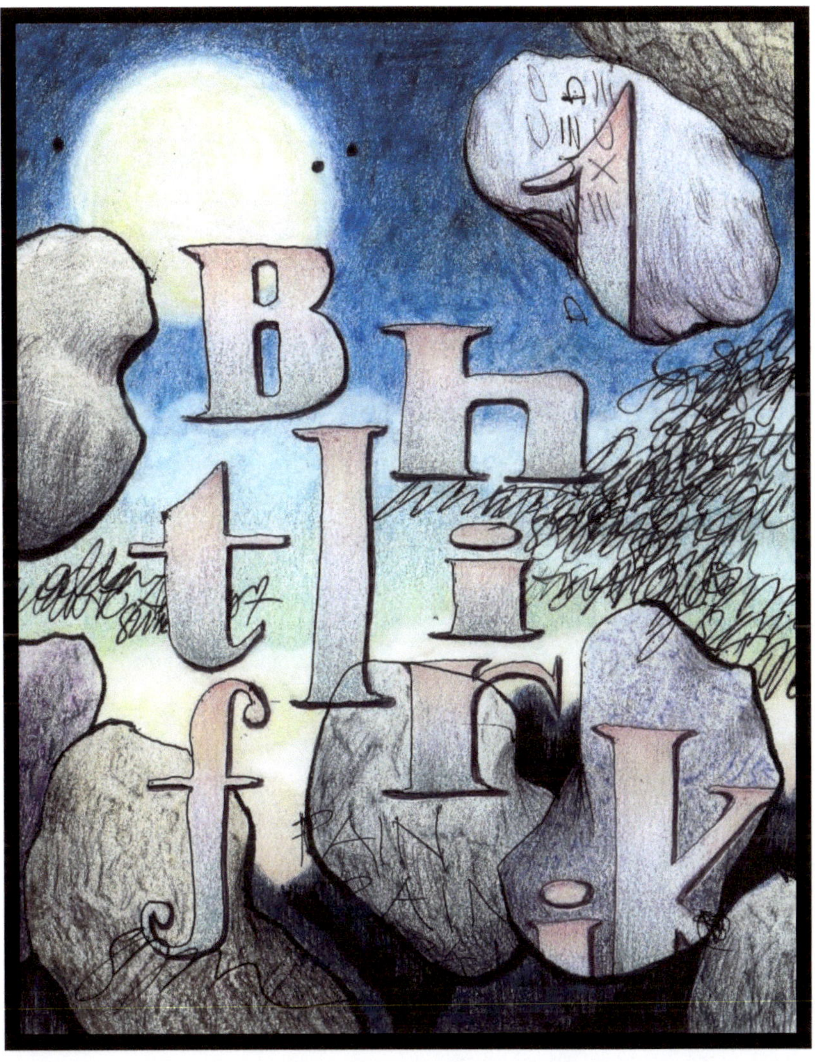
PAIN PAIN

Dreamdate #20 – Easter

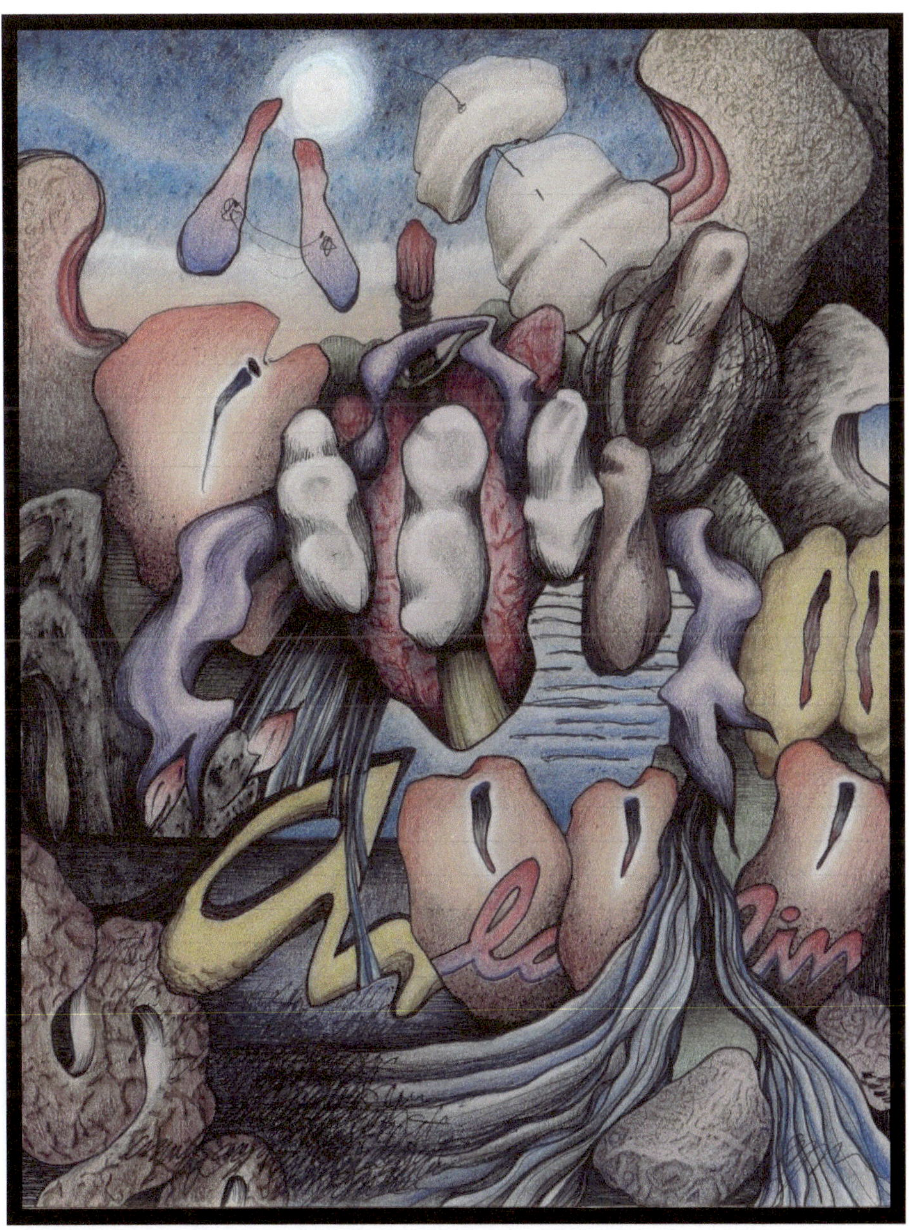

Dreamdate #21 – Wallpaper

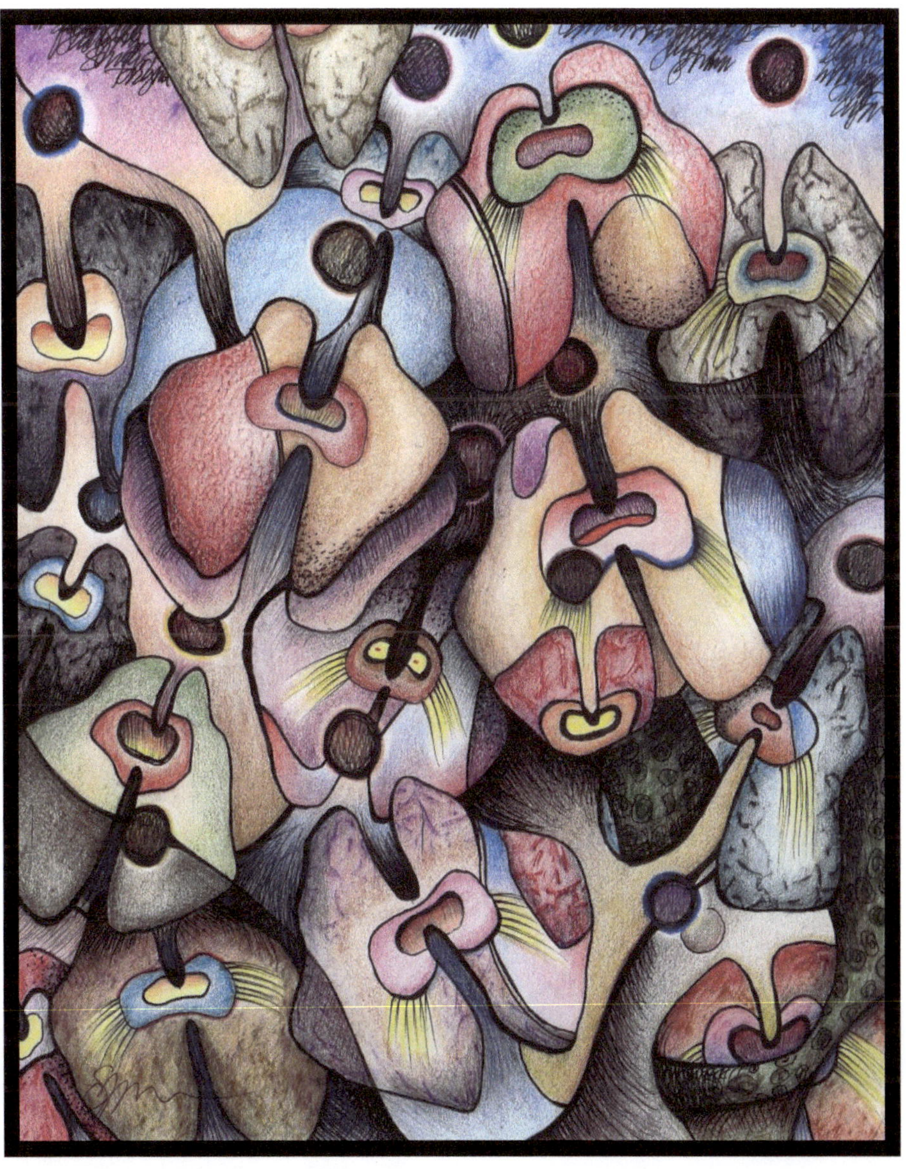

Notes-

ABOUT THE AUTHOR

After growing up in the sprawling metropolis of Tullahoma, TN, Susan studied art in GA. She completed her post-graduate studies in TN, then lived and worked in the ATL for many years. However, in 2007 she had the opportunity (and good sense) to move to NC and is now close enough to the sky and the grassy balds of the southern highlands to feel at home.

She has been scratching out drawings on paper for as long as she can remember. The <u>Alien Spacebaby's Dreambook</u> series of internal landscapes pictured in this book utilize found paper, copy, ink, pencil, and charcoal.